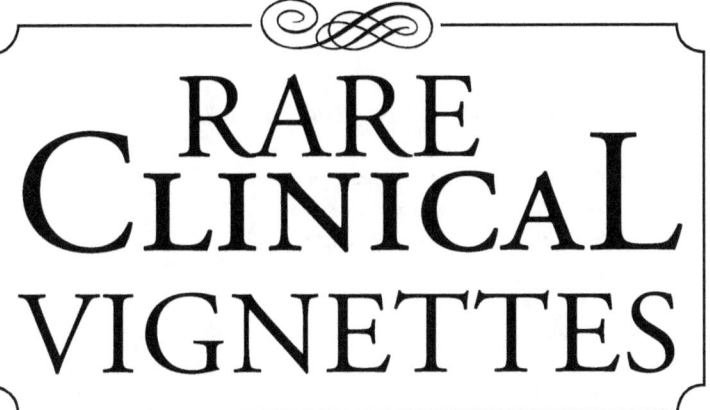

RARE CLINICAL VIGNETTES

ONYECHELA OGBONNA, MD

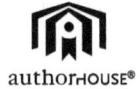

authorHOUSE®

AuthorHouse™
1663 Liberty Drive
Bloomington, IN 47403
www.authorhouse.com
Phone: 1-800-839-8640

The medical information and forum opinion is provided in good faith
to help provide timely care to the sick and needy but should not replace
consultation with your primary care physician or recent medical literature,
because medical information is dynamic and subject to change with time.

Published by AuthorHouse 10/23/2013

ISBN: 978-1-4918-2992-9 (sc)
ISBN: 978-1-4918-2991-2 (e)

Library of Congress Control Number: 2013919273

Any people depicted in stock imagery provided by Thinkstock are models,
and such images are being used for illustrative purposes only.
Certain stock imagery © Thinkstock.

This book is printed on acid-free paper.

Contents

Test Your knowledge

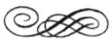

A 56 year old female with Past Medical History of end stage renal disease on dialysis, pancreatic transplant, chronic liver disease of unclear etiology, thrombocytopenia.

She was referred from another hospital for evaluation for possible occult gastroentestinal bleeding to explain her persistent anemia requiring transfusion of packed red blood cell, al most weekly.

She denies gross blood per rectum, black stool, nor coffee ground emesis. No hemotysis.

Work up done, EGD, colonoscopy, bleeding scan and CT abdomen and pelvic, unremarkable.

Consultations include gastroenterology, hematology, nephrology.

video pill cam swallow study of the small intestine was done which made the diagnosis.

What is the diagnosis.

1. **Ormond's Disease**
2. **Mesenteric varices**
3. **Marple syrup urine disease(MSUD)**
4. **Acute Metabolic Encephalopathy**
5. **Polymyositis**
6. **Multiple System Atrophy(MSA)**
7. bleeding diverticulosis of the colon.
8. bleeding esophageal varices
9. intraperitoneal hemorrhage
10. bleeding AAA.
11. slow intracranial hemorrhage
12. dialysis AV shunt related bleeding.
13. Dilutional anemia due to fluid overload as a result of renal failure and ineffective dialysis.

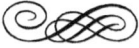

CHAPTER 1

Ormond's Disease as a rare cause of renal failure

Case Report

A 77 year old male with past medical history of hypertension, diabetes, A. fib not on coumadin, renal stones, gout arthritis, Treated Pulmonary TB.

He Presented to ER with chief complains of severe flank pain for 2 weeks sharp, constant, progressive, 9/10, bilateral low back and abdomen, gradual onset, no relieving nor aggravating factors,.

Associated with urinary frequency, burning, and about 20Ib weight loss in 6 months, nausea, joint pain, intermitent cough, loss of appetite

Review of system, social and family history unremarkable

Remarkable physical examination include Positive Bilateral CVA tenderness,

Guaiac negative stool, with tender on prostate palpation

Investigations revealed, Initial BMP showed BUN of 105, cr of 10 consistent with renal failure

EKG Abnormal: Afib

Urineanalysis abnormal showed high wbc

CT chest abd:showed retroperitneal mass, with hydronephrosis, and bilateral lung fibrosis

---

HOSPITAL COURSE

Nephrology consulted and dialysis began temporarily with expectation that ureteral stent will resolve renal failure

Urologist consulted bilateral ureteral stent placed, yet renal functions, did not improved,

Vascular consulted, permecath placed and continue hemodialysis

Oncology consulted, recommended tissue diagnosis

Pulmonary consulted: Patient isolated and AFB, PPD negative.

Retroperitoneal biospy done: no malignant tissue, showed fibrosis with lymphocyte

Final Pathologist Report: sclerotic stroma infiltrated with lymphocytes, stain for acid fast bacilli and amyloid negative, this is consistent with retroperitoneal fibrosis.

DISCUSSION

This disorder has also been referred to as Ormond's disease, periureteritis fibrosa, periureteritis plastica, chronic periureteritis, sclerosing retroperitoneal granuloma, and fibrous retroperitonitis.

Reports describing idiopathic retroperitoneal fibrosis first appeared in the English medical literature in 1948.

CLINICAL PRESENTATION:

The disease presents insidiously, often making the diagnosis difficult. Early symptoms may include a vague, poorly localized pain over the flank, low back, and abdomen, or nonspecific systemic complaints, such as malaise, anorexia, weight loss, moderate pyrexia, nausea, and vomiting

The presence of retroperitoneal fibrosis may be suspected from the characteristic pain but is more often detected as part of the evaluation for urinary tract obstruction or venous or arterial insufficiency.

EPIDERMIOLOGY

Retroperitoneal fibrosis is a rare disease, with an incidence estimated to range from 1:200,000 to 1:500,000 per year and its prevalence is around 1 to 2 per 100,000 inhabitants

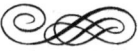

CHAPTER 2

Mesenteric varices as The cause of occult Gastrointestinal bleeding

PRESENTATION OF CASE

A 66-year-old Woman was transferred to this hospital from another facility for further investigation for progressive weakness

She presented to the referring hospital with progressive generalized weakness of about 3months duration that worsened 2 days prior to her admission. She describes the weakness as "whole body weakness" now requiring help for all her activities of daily living.

Remarkable Review of systems: She has noticed intermittent dark stool, but no gross bright red blood rectal bleeding, no hematemesis, no diarrhea, no chest pain, no recent travel.

She has lost over 20 pounds over the last 3 month despite good appetite.

She has a past Medical history of End stage renal disease secondary to uncontrolled diabetes mellitus. She underwent successful living donor renal transplant 2003, placed on immunosuppressive medication, which included cellcept and prednisone.

Her renal function remained stable until July 2011, when She developed acute transplant Kidney rejection, requiring renal replacement therapy, during severe acute illness due to septicemia from septic arthritis, despite aggressive intravenous antibiotics treatment, fluid resuscitation and transplant team intervention. She has been doing well on regular hemodialysis since 2011.

Her Diabetes mellitus has been well controlled after she underwent pancreatic transplant on 2007, taking her immunosuppressive medications regularly.

ON PHYSICAL EXAMINATION

Vitals:Temperature 95.6F, Heart rate 76, Blood pressure 130/58 saturation 98 percent on room air.

General: she is sitting with husband in no apparent distress, awake, oriented to person, time and place, no confusions.

Gen.: - In Respiratory distress, Oriented in time, space, person(x3), orthopnea, alert, depressed.

Head: ATraumatic, Normocephalic,

Eye: Pale conjunctiva, Pupils are reactive to light equally

Ear/ Nose: clear, no abnormalities,.

Mouth/throat: no lesions, has good dentition, no tonsils enlargement, no erythema

Neck:- supple, no JVD, no carotid bruits, lymph nodes. No Thyroid enlargment.

Left ankle trace Edema,

Heart: on inspection deformities, PMI not displaced, no heaves, S1S2 regular, no Murmur no Gallops

Chest: unlabored breathing, On auscultation, clear, no Crackles no, Rubs, Rhonchi, no wheezing.

Abdomen: Post Surgical scar present, Bowel sounds present and normative in 4 quadrant on palpation, hepatomegaly, splenomegaly,- tenderness, - rebound tenderness, no CVA tenderness.

Rectal examination:no hemorrhoid, stool is heme positive

Neuro.: Sensation to Dull sharp, C2- C 12., intact finger to nose, Negative Babinski, Memory and concentration normal. Power equal on all extremities

INVESTIGATIONS:

Laboratory findings:

1. **Hemogram showed low hemoglobin, which improved after transfusion of parked red blood cells**

2. EGD. initial upper endoscopy showed blood clots on gastric body with normal esophagus colonoscopy:showed normal colon,

Repeat EGD:repeat upper endoscopy is normal (no esophageal varies, no duodenal ulcers)

Video capsule endoscopy demonstrated multiple mesenteric(ectopic)varices with stigmata of recent bleeding(red wale sign) of the small bowel.

Transjugular liver biopsy with hepatic pressure measurement, showed normal hepatic pressure

DISCUSSION.

1. Bleeding mesenteric varices. This is a relative rare condition.

IN SUMMARY

Our patient is a 66 year old female with Past medical history of diabetes mellitus off diabetic medication after a successful pancreatic transplant, renal failure on hemodialysis due to failed living donor kidney transplant, chronic idiopathic thrombocytopenia, complaining of generalized weakness and intermittent dark stool diagnosed with iron deficiency anemia, refractory, requiring frequent transfusion of packed red blood cell.

There is high suspicion for occult gastrointestinal bleeding in this case.

She had both upper and lower gastrointestinal endoscopy that is normal.

The likely source of her bleeding will be small intestine, Therefore video capsule endoscopy was done which revealed Mesenteric varices with clinical evidence of recent bleeding.

From Literature review, The presence of mesenteric varices was demonstrated angiographically in 7 patients with portal hypertension. In 4 of these cases the mesenteric varices were the source of lower gastrointestinal bleeding which was successfully controlled by intra-arterial infusion of vasopressin.

Data from the Third National Health and Nutrition Examination Survey (NHANES III; 1988 to 1994) indicated that iron deficiency anemia was present in 1 to 2 percent of adults.

Overt blood loss such as hematemesis, melena, hemoptysis, severe menorrhagia, and gross hematuria not difficult for the clinician to recognize, often based on history alone.

Occult bleeding, on the other hand, may be difficult diagnosis to make. This usually occurs via the gastrointestinal tract in men. Other causes to consider are repeated voluntary blood donations, the post-operative setting in which blood loss greatly exceeds the amount of blood transfused, or iatrogenic anemia due to repeated and massive blood drawing in the course of workup of a complicated medical condition in admitted patients.

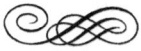

CHAPTER 3

Marple syrup urine disease is a rare metabolic cause of altered mental status

Case Report

A 37 yo old female was brought to the emergency room after her friend noticed that she was disoriented and yelling uncontrollably in the middle

of the street. The Patients friend says that the patient acts that way whenever she becomes noncompliant with her dietary restriction. The onset of the confusion was subacute, lasting a few days.

Past medical history was significant of a previous episode of confusion, that required admission to Mount Sinai medical center.

A peritoneal dialysis was done to remove very high level of toxic metabolic products of branched chain amino acid.

Physical examination were unremarkable except that she had auditory and visual hallucinations and talks to everyone in sign.

Patient had a history of being traumatized during the 9/11 event at The World Trade Center so she constantly talked about it during physical exam.

Investigations:Most of her laboratory findings were unremarkable including normal Complete blood count, basic metabolic profile, hepatic panel, head CT, toxicology screen.

Two samples of amino acid level were sent to quest laboratory and to Mount Sinai Laboratory.

Hospital Course

She was admitted, began IV fluids, Dextrose 5% in water.

The maple syrup urine Disease.

formula special diet was administered. Also food high in Leucine, such as banana was strictly avoided.

The response was rather slow, so Specialist was, Mount Sinai Metabolic doctor was contacted. specific investigations, for MSUD was ordered. Result, the leucine level, as normal and concluded that this episode of confusion was not due to metabolic intoxication.

Psychiatrist consulted

Subsequently the patient was evaluated by psychiatrist with impression of psychosis, haldol 0.5mg was recommended for agitations. The patient responded, returned to baseline, and was discharged, to follow up with metabolic Doctor and Psychiatrist.

Discussion

Marple syrup urine disease is a rare metabolic cause of altered mental status. MSUD, also called branched-chain ketonuria, was reported by Menkes et al in 1954, in a family who lost 4 infants within the first 3 months of their lives because of a neuro-degenerative disorder with urine odor resembling maple syrup (burned sugar)

Branch. Chain Ketoac. dehyd

Deficiency of the BCKD complex, which catalyzes the decarboxylation of the alpha-keto acids of leucine, isoleucine, and valine to their respective branched-chain acyl-CoAs, to yield acetyl-CoA, acetoacetate, and succinyl-CoA. Accumulation of the keto acids of these 3 amino acids leads to encephalopathy and progressive neurodegeneration. Maple Syrup Urine Disease occurs 1 out of 185, 000 births in the United States.

Diagnostic Dilemma

Patients with Maple Syrup Urine Disease (MSUD) usually present with episodes of confusion during periods of metabolic intoxication.

However, in rare cases the confusion may be a manifestation of underlying psychiatric illness and could pose a diagnostic dilemma

Leucine is neurotoxic

Leucine - causes neurological manifestations such as confusion, seizures, etc

Isoleucine - gives maple syrup odor

CONCLUSION

Occasionally, mental state changes in a patient with Maple Syrup urine Disease may be a manifestation of an underlying psychiatric illness. It is not always due to metabolic intoxication from high levels of branched chain amino acids. This may lead to a diagnostic dilemma.

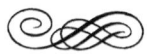

CHAPTER 4

Acute Metabolic Encephalopathy due to high ammonia Level in A Patient without Liver Disease

Case Report:

The patient is an 89-year-old male with past medical history of recent GI bleeding, status post EGD and colonoscopy, history of BPH, compression fracture of L1, history of peripheral neuropathy, was brought into the ED with acute confusion, disorientation, and encephalopathy with more of delirium in the evening time. He has history of social alcohol use but not diagnosed with Liver cirrhosis nor known liver disease.

Hospital Course

He was admitted and had investigations done, which included CT of the head, which showed no acute pathology. He also had an MRI of the brain done, which did not reveal any acute pathology. So, ammonia level was found out to be elevated and he was began on lactulose and his symptoms have resolved and he is feeling much better. He has anemia due to acute on chronic blood loss and the blood work has remarkably improved on iron treatment. The patient has made a remarkable improvement on oral Lactulose solution to reduce ammonia level and omeprazole to control gastrointestinal bleeding and is mental back to his baseline, able to carry out his activities of daily living with minimal family support.

Discussion:

Causes of high ammonia Level, In adults, vary and can include kidney or liver damage, drug and alcohol abuse, and gastrointestinal bleeding.

Our patient above had a recent Gastrointestinal bleeding, which is likely the best explanation for his high ammonia level, which is highly suggestive of continues slow bleeding

High ammonia level is typically a progressive condition. At its onset, may not notice any symptoms at all, or only mild symptoms. As the disease worsens, you may experience more symptoms or symptoms of increased severity. Including

- Confusion or agitations
- Fatigue(Weakness (loss of strength)
- Loss of appetite
- Nausea with or without vomiting
- Falls
- Worsening symptoms in patients with Dementia or sun downing
- Change in level of consciousness or alertness, such as passing out or unresponsiveness
- Changes in mood, personality or behavior

Treatment options for High ammonia Level, Depends on the cause of the condition, our Patient in the clinical case responded well to Lactulose oral solution which reduced his ammonia level and taking omeprazole to prevent gastrointestinal bleeding.

In more serious cases, however, treatment is necessary because the buildup of ammonia in the bloodstream can have serious consequences. Treatment for elevated blood ammonia level is aimed at removing toxic body waste, such as ammonia, from the bloodstream. This can be accomplished through use of medications, dialysis or, in very serious cases, organ transplant depending on clinical situation.

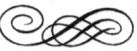

CHAPTER 5

Polymyositis as a very rare Initial Presentation of HIV

Case Report:

A 57 year old male presented to ER with chief complain of bilateral weakness for 2 years which has progressively worsened over 3 weeks, initially had difficulty to walk few block, limited by leg weakness, not pain which progressed to not able to get out of bed, falls when attempting to get up. weakness is generalized and symmetrical but more pronounced on lower extremity than upper, associated with mild, intermittent muscle tenderness, symptoms are not relieved by rest.

Review Of Systems

Denies rash, fever, slurred speak or stroke like symptom, no recent trauma, statin, colchicines, steroid, visual complains., weight loss, Positive past social history of homosexual contacts, drug use.

Patient has multiple medical problems which includes, seizure disorder, hepatitis C, depression diabetes, hypothyroidism, emphysema hydrocephalus status post ventricular peritoneal shunt, and recently diagnosed polymyoisitis confirmed by muscle biopsy report from private doctor for which he has been receiving intravenous immunoglobulins for about 4 months with good response, but due to financial reasons was not able to continue during the last 3 weeks before presentation to use was never on steroid, not tested for HIV, not yet worked up for malignancy. medications included, synthroid, Zoloft, dilantin, repaglinid., albutrol.

Physical examination were unremarkable except for bilateral symmetrical proximal muscle weakness in both upper and lower extremity, reduced strength 4/5 upper and 3/5 lower, associated with mild tenderness on palpation, no fasciculation, atrophy, with intact sensations.

No rash(Gottron's sign, heliotrope rash, mechanic's hand)

The above physical/motor findings fluctuate rapidly from not able to get up, to a brief episode of ablity to walk to nursing station

His laboratory findings were remarkable for high CK initially 2480 later trended down to 320, positive antismooth muscle antibody with titer 1:80, anti Jo less than 1.0, Sjogreen negative,. TSH low at 0.23, high ESR 70.

THE HOSPITAL COURSE

Rheumatology was consulted, they recommended intravenous solumedrol, calcium, vitamin D, and to follow up CK, level. Our Patient responded dramatically with improved muscle strength, He began to ambulate, The solumedrol was later switched to oral prednisone.

Subsequently, The patient was appropriately counseled for HIV testing to which he consented to, initial test was reported as positive which was later confirmed by the Western blot. CD4 count 224.

Based on this new diagnosis HIV myopathy was considered so Infectious disease was consulted, recommended to continue current effective management and to follow up in immunology clinic

During the hospital course, the patient continued to improve on oral medications, ambulating well, very grateful and agreed to discharge and follow up plan at the immunology and rheumatology clinic. He was discharged.

DISCUSSION:

To our knowledge based on literature review, Since 1986 there has been only 2 cases of Polymyosistis as the initial presentation of HIV.

Establishing the cause of myalgia is crucial in the management of HIV patient. Whereas uncomplicated myalgia associated with viremia such as HIV and fibromyagia typically requires symptomatic treatment, myopathies associated with HIV or its treatment desearve special consideration because these disorders are potentially disabling and life threatening.

1. Polymyositis and dermatomyositis - Autoimmunity (The original Bohan and Peter criteria, formulated in 1975, included the following features [3]:
   - Symmetric proximal muscle weakness
   - Typical rash of DM, which was the only distinguishing feature between DM and PM
   - Elevated serum muscle enzymes
   - Myopathic changes on electromyography
   - Characteristic muscle biopsy abnormalities and the absence of histopathologic signs of other myopathies
2. Drug effect - AZT and didanosine
3. Secondary neoplasm - Lymphoma and Kaposi sarcoma
4. Myasthenic syndrome and chronic fatigue - Autoimmune
5. Rhabdomyolysis - Opportunistic infection, HIV, didanosine, lamivudine

TREATMENT

- Polymyositis and dermatomyositis improve with steroids.
- In AZT myopathy, discontinue AZT or decrease dose and begin administration of an alternative drug. Muscle enzymes and strength return to normal 1-2 months after the drug is discontinued.
- Carnitine has been shown to prevent development of this condition and progression of AZT myopathy when already present.

- In didanosine-induced rhabdomyolysis, discontinue didanosine.
- Myasthenic syndrome is treated similar to myasthenia gravis, with steroids, intravenous immunoglobulin G, pyridostigmine, and HAART.

For HIV-associated polymyositis, pulsed IV methylprednisolone is preferable to long-term oral prednisone to minimize immunosuppression.

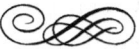

CHAPTER 6

Multiple System Atrophy(MSA)

Case Report

- 53 year-old alcoholic male presented to the emergency room with altered mental status. Last drink was 1 day prior to admission. He is an ex-smoker with history of Dementia.

Remarkable Physical Examination, findings include:He was oriented only to person, not in distress, had resting tremor of right arm, which improved with use and the patient was able to control it voluntarily for a while. His gait was Unstable, positive for Orthostatic hypotension.

Positive findings in Investigations include, hyponatremia, Head CT revealed sinusitis, Abnormal EKG with ST changes, Elevated troponin, Abnormal Cosyntropin test, Low serum osmolality, High urine sodium osmolality

Hospital Course

- During Treatment for NSTEMI, adrenal insufficiency and for alcohol withdrawal, Hyponatremia worsens, associated with Worsening altered mental status, so he was, Transferred to ICU, consultations was done, Endocrinology advised to continue fluid restriction and start sodium tablets. Management of NSTEMI continued, Pancytopenia and fever developed, which improved after discontinuing Plavix.

- Mental status, pancytopenia and hyponatremia improved, then.
- When the Patient's mental state improved enough to provide detailed history he stated, that his resting tremor has been present for 1 year and was associated with unsteady gait and dizziness. Neurology consultant finds Parkingsonian features, suggested a trial of levodopa/carbidopa which did not substantially improve symptoms.
- Subsequently, Patient became stable and was transferred to Elmhurst hospital center for cardiac catheterization

CONCLUSION:

- Our Patient had the clinical features of MSA:
  - *Autonomic dysfunction* – Dizziness, adrenal dysfunction, hyponatremia.
  - *Parkinsonism* – tremors at rest, rigidity of muscles, slowness in moving (confirmed by neurologist).
  - *Cerebellar dysfunction* – ataxia, maintaining balance, and coordinating voluntary movements.
  - Prognosis is generally worse than with idiopathic PD (Parkinson disease)as there is no effective treatment making accurate diagnosis vital for their management.

DISCUSSION

- Definition:MSA is a progressive, idiopathic, degenerative process beginning in adulthood. Patients present with various degrees of parkinsonism, autonomic failure, cerebellar dysfunction and pyramidal signs that are poorly responsive to levodopa or dopamine agonists. Glial cytoplasmic inclusions and a neuronal multisystem degeneration are the pathologic hallmarks of this clinically variable disorder

  o In 2003, the Movement Disorders Society Scientific Issues Committee Report revised the diagnostic criteria for MSA and subdivided it into 2 categories:
    - MSA-P: predominant Parkinsonian features
    - MSA-C: prominent cerebellar dysfunction features

  o Patients with idiopathic PD are distinguished from patients with MSA by the lack of autonomic and cerebellar features as well as by their response to levodopa/carbidopa.

Patients with MSA typically do not substantially benefit from trials of levodopa/carbidopa.

Introduction

The symptoms experienced in Multiple System Atrophy (MSA) come from the loss of nerve cells in the nervous system. MSA is most likely to be confused with idiopathic Parkingsons Disease (PD).

- Symptoms are grouped into three main categories:

  Autonomic dysfunction – urinary incontinence, erectile dysfunction, orthostatic hypotension, fainting, constipation

  Parkinsonism – tremors at rest, rigidity of muscles, slowness in moving

  Cerebellar dysfunction – ataxia, maintaining balance, and coordinating voluntary movements.

Epidemiology

As MSA is frequently under-recognized, the exact incidence of MSA is not known. Researchers estimated the average annual incidence of MSA was 3 cases per 100,000 population. It is estimated that 3-10% of patients with PD actually have MSA-P. The disease has a male predominance.

About the Author

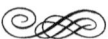

Onyechela Ogbonna, MD is a medical doctor with great clinical experience.

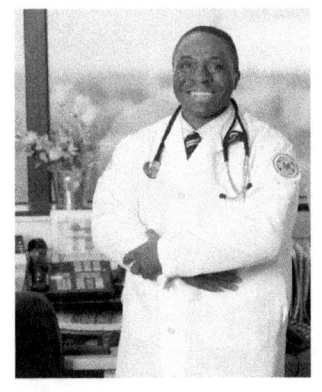

He is the Author of the Book " The Best Clinical Guide"

He is board certified in internal medicine. He completed medical training at the Mount Sinai School of Medicine in Queens, New York.

His current clinical duty includes direct care to thousands of patients and supervising medical residents, students, nurses, physician assistants, and APRNs. He does medical consultations in the emergency department for management of complex conditions. He advises patients and their families on health-related issues.

He is a hospital physician based in Hartford Hospital, a major referral hospital in Hartford, Connecticut.

About the Book

Rare Clinical Vignettes is a collection of Clinical Cases.

The Book is Based on True Life Experiences, Rare Medical conditions and Diagnostic Dilemma, Including Ormond's Disease as a rare cause of renal failure.

Mesenteric varices as a Rare cause of occult Gastrointestinal bleeding. Marple syrup urine disease(MSUD) is a rare metabolic cause of altered mental status in Adults, Acute Metabolic Encephalopathy due to high ammonia Level in A Patient without Liver Disease.

Polymyositis as a very rare Initial Presentation of HIV

Multiple System Atrophy(MSA) in a Patient with Parkinson's Syndrome.